HOW TO PREVENT AND SURVIVE FOOD-BORNE DISEASES

ALLERGIES AND INFECTIOUS DISEASES

Additional books in this series can be found on Nova's website under the Series tab.

Additional E-books in this series can be found on Nova's website under the e-books tab.

HOW TO PREVENT AND SURVIVE FOOD-BORNE DISEASES

ALCIDES TRONCOSO

Department of Microbiology and Infectious Diseases,
School of Medicine-Buenos Aires University,
Department of Food-Borne Diseases,
Belgrano University, Buenos Aires, Argentina

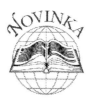

Nova Science Publishers, Inc.
New York

For permission to use material from this book please contact us:
Telephone 631-231-7269; Fax 631-231-8175
Web Site: http://www.novapublishers.com

LIBRARY OF CONGRESS CATALOGING-IN-PUBLICATION DATA

ISBN: 978-1-61942-683-2

Published by Nova Science Publishers, Inc. † New York

WITHDRAWN

CONTENTS

PREFACE

Food-borne diseases are one of the major threats for public health. This happens because of the presence of pathogenic microorganisms in any raw food, mainly in fresh fruits and vegetables, dairy products and meat, among others. In order to reduce the diseases related to the consumption of these foods, it is required the collaboration of the official organisms that are in charge of the population' health care, of the food industry, health institutions and consumers. There is no doubt that the surveillance of the food contamination requires a many-sided view, which includes all the entities involved in the food chain, from the farm to the table. Moreover, a properly coordinated strategy is required, in which all the control organisms that are in charge of the foods' harmlessness and safety are present.

In the industrialized countries, the current situation has brought questions to the consumers as regards the foods' harmlessness, as well as distrust of the existing food control systems. As a consequence, it is urgent to claim to the health ministers a great political willingness to make efforts in order to grant the foods' harmlessness. Even though it is known partially, the morbidity hidden burden and the current data are, in fact, alarming. Just by analysing what is happening and the uncertainty, we can realise that once the diseases is acquired, one does not know who to pray. As regards this, it is worth highlighting that in the underdeveloped countries the food-borne diseases burden is clear and endemic. This unfortunately happens because of the consumers' lack of awareness as well as because of politicians' carelessness, as there is usually little political willingness to properly deal with these matters, which means correctly doing the correct thing. The gap between developed and underdeveloped countries is not only economical; it is mainly intellectual and moral. The people like me, who have "zero tolerance" to apathy and indifference, may want the things to be different. The fact of setting up alliances between industrialized countries and developing countries will allow us to benefit from the previous and current experiences with the aim of promoting the foods' harmlessness at a national and international level.

The aim of this book is to use this opportunity to work seeking for the safest foods for everyone, as well as to pass on my own experiences and my colleagues'· experiences, which come from the thorough study of specialized publications. As regards this, this book has follows these steps: 1) I analyzed what I know, 2) I looked for gaps in knowledge, 3) I criticised stated commitments, claiming and demanding rigor in the health authorities from the countries that often, if not always, have a special system to hide the problems in public health by pretending that such problems do not exist, and 4) I paid attention to inconsistency and contradictions, as well as to the shown conclusions. This is the great merit of this book, but it is also its limit. One doesn't write to be read. How can one give vitality to each of these chapters, each with its own "atomic weight" if there are no readers, the ones who are destined to decode the symbols? One writes for this, and only for this; not to amaze or to have "success", because if a book belongs of the ones who remain, the aim is achieved and the author can be "deleted". I hope that the teachings I want to transmit are so simple that everyone may be pleased because they completely understand them. In short, I do not consider that the researches about diseases related to foods are finished, and this book shows my wish to go on reflecting on and setting up new ideas, while some others pay attention to this problem. A discerning palate is not necessary to notice that avoiding this difficult project would be equivalent to assuming the responsibility of cutting short a work continuity that constantly points at the future.

Prof. Alcides Troncoso,
M.D., Ph.D.

FOREWORD

Given that microorganisms are everywhere, they naturally appear in plants and animals. A small percentage of these microorganisms is pathogenic and, therefore, requires control measures. It could be thought that finding a microbial etiological agent in a food could be very useful. But, maybe, the detection in foods of microorganisms will only be tackled when an outbreak occurs.

The investigation of outbreaks and routine monitoring presupposes many different types of priorities. When persons are already ill, the relatively high cost of detecting a virus in food samples may be acceptable, especially if litigation is foreseen. Nevertheless, an outbreak of hepatitis A, which affects several people, will probably only be identified four weeks or more after the contaminated food has been consumed, and therefore, it is possible that no samples are found of the relevant foods for analysis.

Consequently, the analysis of foods in order to know if they are contaminated, with the hope of preventing human illnesses, has special problems. The costs will possibly exceed the demonstrable benefits. On the other hand, as most viruses and many bacteria are transmitted through the fecal-oral cycle, it is possible that one or another agent is present in food, due to fecal contamination. In spite of how ingenious the methods developed for detecting microorganisms transmitted through foods are, none can be considered for routine use.

It is imperative to highlight the necessity of guaranteeing the total microbial innocuousness of foods. On the other hand, various sequential factors are associated with food-transmitted diseases (FTD). These are: (1) a pathogen must get to the food; (2) it must survive there until it is consumed, (3) in some cases, it must proliferate until reaching infectious levels or producing toxins, and (4) the person who eats the food must be sensitive to the ingested levels.

When good handling practices are not employed, food contamination can occur in any step of the food chain—during its production, processing, distribution and/or manufacturing as well as in its sale. *Everyone in the alimentary system, from the person producing the food to that who prepares it, plays a significant role in its innocuousness*, including the activities amply defined as "food handling."

Several studies have proven that some people consider that home is the place where food innocuousness problems are less likely to appear. On the contrary, epidemiologic studies carried out in the United States indicate that sporadic cases and small home outbreaks cover the majority of the cases of food-transmitted diseases. Botulism, campilobacteriosis and listeriosis are frequently caused by a bad handling of foods at home.

People involved in each one of the alimentary system sectors need to understand the reasons why it is necessary to maintain a pro-active control regarding food innocuousness. These reasons are: (1) microorganisms are everywhere and are found in raw agricultural products, (2) pathogens may survive minimum conservation treatments, (3) just before its consumption, human beings may introduce pathogens in foods during their production, processing, distribution and/or manufacturing, (4) depending on individual sensitivity, food-transmitted diseases may range from mild to very serious and lethal or may produce chronic complications.

Several changes occurred in society that contributed to microbiological challenges. Few people happen to express their worries with respect to food innocuousness; in fact, there is an increase in the use of easy preparation foods and diminishment of the degree of training received by people regarding adequate food handling, which may have caused suppositions concerning food innocuousness and the subsequent complacent attitude. It is a fact that a *contaminated food may be indistinguishable from a non-contaminated food*. These changes may result in neither children nor young adults learning the basic principles for preparing foods.

The majority of individuals do not know that inadequate practices in food handling may increase the risk of acquiring diseases. These mistakes are responsible for the great majority of diseases transmitted by home food. All people should be conscious of the control that is necessary in their own kitchens for preventing food-transmitted diseases. They also need to know how important the food handling practices are—acquisition, storage and preparation, how to serve food and keep leftovers—and how these practices affect innocuousness of food.

Education through specific programs addressed to increase knowledge in health professionals is the key instrument for preventing the risks of food-transmitted diseases. In order to train the public in general to make well-informed decisions about food innocuousness—decisions that affect their health—the educational efforts that the interdisciplinary team makes must provide precise reasons regarding the necessity of supervising to be certain that food-handling practices are appropriate.

To achieve food microbial innocuousness is an increasing concern, particularly when you take into consideration that *contamination may be irreversible, actually, washing vegetables does not eliminate pathogens such as Enterohemorragic Escherichia coli (EHEC)*. Some foods that are consumed fresh, as are "all the greens," are very possibly contaminated, maybe due to the fact that the great majority of them are prone to being manhandled during harvest or because certain characteristics of the plant surfaces facilitate the microbial penetration; therefore, *it should be assumed that "all the greens" may be dangerous, even when there does not exist substantial evidence that proves that it is a threat to human health.*

Contamination is the rule and not the exception in a world where microorganisms' vast spreading offers them many opportunities to be transmitted through foods that are consumed. Even worse, many professionals who are responsible for "health care" continue promoting fresh fruit and vegetable consumption without having reasonable knowledge about how consumption of a contaminated food may trigger a serious adverse consequence for health or, even worse, death.

The agents and clinical presentations' spectrum is ample and includes diseases that have long incubation periods such as hepatitis A and Lysteriosis and diseases such as botulism and ciguatera (fish poisoning), in which gastrointestinal symptoms are not the relevant part of the clinic presentation. Gastrointestinal infection due to *Enterohemorrhagic E coli* or *Campylobacter* may be followed by two threatening sequelae, HUS and Guillain Barre Syndrome, respectively. Some people may wonder "if something is happening" with food contamination. It could be thought that this would be a typical problem of poor countries, where hygienic conditions are appalling. But this is not so, since the incidents of alimentary intoxications during the last years in Europe as well as in the United States have been alarming.

Taking into account that for some age groups certain pathogens offer a far greater danger for human life than others and may cause serious and potentially deadly diseases, health care promoters should advise about which foods may put at risk the most vulnerable patients. Knowledge of these dangers offers the opportunity for advising which foods should be avoided by consumers, so as to reduce the risk of becoming infected with a disease.

Zero tolerance for bacterial infection implies considering inclusion of "radiation on the table." Although radiation is one of the food processing methods that have been studied most thoroughly and extensively, its use, however, is still controversial. Innocuousness is the most important factor. Although innocuousness has been well established *(there is unanimous agreement within the scientific community),* there are some occasional questions. But there is no consistent and reproducible study that shows or suggests that *the consumption of an irradiated food implies a risk increase for the consumer.* It is necessary to deny the mistakes generally made about irradiation, particularly the idea that foods turn radioactive. From the analysis of the vast amount of scientific data offered by around 500 references in specialized journals, it emerges that foods irradiated in accordance with a technologically useful dose interval so as to achieve the foreseen microbiological target are considered innocuous, healthy and adequate from a nutritional point of view.

For example, no one could call into question that *E coli* 0157: H7 can cause death. Irradiated meat does not. In conclusion, food irradiation risks are unknown simply because scientists—after four decades of investigations—have not found any. This is a sufficiently sound argument against the known risks of contracting a food-transmitted bacterial disease.

Over and over, microorganisms take advantage of any minor opening and opportunity for causing their fearsome effects. It is as if they had an intelligence of their own, a capacity for responding with weapons superior to those employed against them. *Their smallness and invisibility not only does not obstruct but encourages its effects to be far terrible with a fundamental purpose, that of ending human life, which is its greater enemy. The possibility of implying foods in the appearance or reappearance in human beings of microbial threats is immense. It is the revenge of the viruses and the bacteria.*

Constant epidemiologic surveillance is the tool for guaranteeing good health. Whilst the members of a health team may have different perspectives regarding some of the data and recommendations conveyed in this ambitious information compendium that deals with FTD prevention, those differences are an essential component and a characteristic feature of this project.

We have decided to accept this obligation. In sharing our knowledge and our doubts, our questions and our answers and our determination for defending the dignity and value of human life, we are taking a very important step forward.

When we started to share our knowledge in this manuscript rough draft and wrote the committed assigned chapters, we were anticipating that, in addition, we would learn what was mutually shared. As health care professionals working within a group of investigators and professors from two Argentine Universities—the Microbiology and Infectious Diseases Department at the University of Buenos Aires and the Food-Transmitted Diseases Department of the University of Belgrano—we assumed a commitment to volunteer valuable and useful resources for the Health Ministries and hospital directors who value and respect human life and who must make decisions to protect it. This book is especially intended for the general public as well as for non-specialized health professionals who are interested in completing their training with regard to FTD (physicians, nutritionists, sanitary agents, epidemiologists, etc.). With this purpose, necessary tools are discussed in detail for all those who have the responsibility of protecting population at risk of acquiring food-transmitted bacterial diseases. Beyond question, the training and documentation that health professionals must have regarding the means for preventing, controlling or eliminating microbial risks associated with human food should be clear, consistent and scientifically sustainable.

It should be explicitly stated that we present this book as an invitation to involve our colleagues in the topic of food-transmitted diseases. We also want to encourage organization and opinion leaders in two particular matters: re-awakening a call for being practical and specific, and in applying scientific knowledge whilst answering urgent health problems that must be faced, and we reject doing so in an abstract and speculative way.

As the main individual responsible for this book, I want to highlight the collaboration of Etienne Cardwell, whose long hours spent reviewing the book I can attest to. I am grateful for the critical reading Isabella Garcia-Moreno did of the book and Constanza Lopez Meller for his elementary good sense, which gave way to the elimination of two chapters that were expendable in view of the proposed goals. Among the Argentine collaborators, I want to emphasize the valuable work of Mariela Tornese and of Celeste Seley.

I must not forget to mention the René Barón Foundation (RBF) and its President, in particular, Engineer Mr. Carlos Baron Biza, who sponsored the first book on food-transmitted disease prevention carried out in South America. For more than 30 years, RBF has been the cultural sponsor of several national and international non-profit scientific projects, among them, the book that was the manuscript on which the current English version is based.

Alcides Troncoso,
MD, PhD

Chapter 1

BOTULISM

Texas, United States of America, 1993. An epidemic affects 17 persons. They showed nausea, mouth dryness and, strikingly, blurred double vision. When they attended an emergency ward, it was detected that all had in common the fact that they had consumed a few hours before a food known as "skordalia," which is manufactured using a potato base and a packaged cheese sauce. This sauce had been prepared with boiled potatoes, which after they were cooked had been hermetically sealed with aluminum foil and kept at room temperature in an oxygen-lacking environment for several days.

A most dangerous venom produced by the *Clostridium botulinum* bacteria, which is harmless if found in an air-exposed food, was the cause of the Texas epidemic outbreak. In fact, a person can consume, with no risk at all, foods having the bacteria spore. However, in anaerobiosis conditions (e.g., in the absence of oxygen), the spore produces a potent neurotoxin that is the most deadly known venom.

Botulism was first described by European sausage consumers in the XVIII century and is related with commercial canned foods, which provoked epidemics during the XIX and XX centuries, before the standard deactivation methods of spores lodged in tins was perfected by means of industrial sterilization. Around the beginning of the XX century, the number of outbreaks produced by commercial canned foods diminished, but home-canned foods have become the main botulism cause, not only of sporadic cases, but also of outbreaks, including those taking place at restaurants.

In Argentina, the majority of cases have been provoked by the consumption of foods (asparagus, pickled or marinated foods—known as escabeche), which were stored in homemade containers. In January 1998, an outbreak occurred in Buenos Aires; it affected several bus drivers. Of 11 people who had consumed the food, 9 of them (82%) developed the disease. It was detected as botulinum neurotoxin type A, and the food associated with the outbreak was *matambre* (rolled and stuffed meat). Said food had been cooked in water at a 78 to 80 °C temperature for four hours, sealed in a plastic bag and inadequately refrigerated, which contributed to the survival, germination and synthesis of the neurotoxins, which caused the disease: *C botulinum*.

It is important to emphasize that foods that contain the botulinic toxin may have an absolutely normal aspect and taste; this means that a healthy food is indistinguishable by its aspect, taste and smell from a dangerous one.

What is Botulism?

The botulinic toxin is a protein produced by the *Clostridium botulinum* bacteria; it is found around the world in soil and in marine sediment forming spores that allow it to survive in nature. It is harmless in that state. But in foods placed under conditions lacking oxygen, the bacterial spores can germinate, multiply and start producing the toxin.

There exist seven different immunological toxins. They are designated with letters A to G, and three of them are those that most affect the human being: types A and B have world distribution; E type is found in fish.

When ingesting foods carrying the preformed toxin, it arrives to the place where the nervous stimulus transmission is produced—the neurons or nerve cells—thus producing a paralysis of upper and lower extremities and of respiratory muscles, which is 100% deadly, if not treated.

Where is Botulism Found?

The home, handmade bottling or canning of foods as well as pickling (asparagus, tomato, peppers, cheese with onion, garlic, viscacha) in (plastic or glass) sealed containers creates the anaerobic conditions (without oxygen) that allow the germination of the *Clostridium botulinum* spores.

Traditional foods, especially those foods that are fermented such as fish, roe (fish eggs), viscacha, beaver and whale, have caused botulism, chiefly in Alaska. Foods are prepared in such a way that permits fermentation at room temperature, and they are usually consumed without previous cooking.

Meat, in particular *pork*, may be a source of botulism. In the intestine of this animal, spores and vegetative forms of *C botulinum* are present, and if they cross the intestinal mucosa, they arrive to the circulatory stream, reaching striated muscles where, under favorable circumstances, spores germinate and vegetative forms multiply and synthesize the neurotoxin. The spores' and the vegetative forms' arrival to circulation is favored by several circumstances:

- If the animal slaughter is performed without subjecting it to a 24- hour previous fasting.
- Tiredness and extreme fatigue of the animals to be slaughtered increase the permeability of intestinal walls and permit spores and toxins to reach more easily the systemic circulation. In addition, these "tired meats," give birth to a higher pH (alkaline or less acid), which sweats easily and therefore does not retain the salt that acts, in products such as cured ham, as a stop to *C. botulinum* germination.
- In case of badly bled meats, there exists a higher risk of producing botulinic neurotoxins in meats that are destined to the curing process.
- In case of late evisceration, an excessive contact may occur between meat and the intestinal contents with an increasing risk of bacteria contaminating the meat.
- In cases of meat coming from pigs that are sick due to different kinds of illnesses, the correct salting of the pieces chosen for preparing ham prevents the disease.

Botulinic neurotoxins have been detected in several meat products such as ham, smoked cuts and Frankfurt-like sausages vacuum-packaged in plastic bags. There is no doubt that vacuum packaging is dangerous if the product does not require a previous heat-up before it is consumed. A meat product that is involved with a certain frequency in botulism cases is home-cured ham (incorrectly prepared), which usually contains B neurotoxin such as it has been documented in Portugal, Spain, France and Poland.

Bacteria habitat in fish is located in the intestinal tract and excrements. Numerous botulism outbreaks associated with fish prepared in varied ways such as: salted, smoked, fermented or preserved. Botulism outbreaks due to fermented fish, which is prepared at home for its preservation among Alaska and Canada natives, have been recorded and have also occurred through uneviscerated salted fish (*ribyetz*) a Jewish traditional recipe. Botulism associated with traditional recipes based on uneviscerated fish was also documented in preparations such as Egyptian *fasikh* and *kapchunka*, which come from Eastern Europe. The 1992 E botulism outbreak caused by *mohola*, a traditional Egyptian fish salt-cured that was bought in a New Jersey market, falls within this category and was the first communicated outbreak associated with commercial fish that was incorrectly handled. Three cases of type B botulism, which happened in 1990, in Hawaii, were caused by a kind of *palani* fish. This outbreak was unusual because the fish was bought fresh in a retail establishment but was insufficiently cooked. The serious disease seemed to be associated with the consumption of insufficiently cooked fish intestines. Since then, the sale of uneviscerated fish has been banned in many places.

In Alaska, type E toxin is responsible for more than 85% of botulism cases as many of the traditional local native foods, amongst which are included salmon's head, whale grease, skin and oil of seals and roe are prepared by fermentation under conditions that may encourage the germination and growth of the neurotoxin. To eat dead whale grease, as was described in those outbreaks, shows respect towards tradition; however, storing in grease of that kind or of another kind in hermetically sealed plastic bags, which may create an anaerobic environment, is a modern discovery. The use of hermetic containers for storing and fermenting traditional foods is partly considered responsible for the increase in the incidence of botulism in different parts of the world.

In infants under one year old, a common botulism source is exposure to spores found in the ground, honey consumption or the administration of homemade tisanes or "herbal homemade teas" (such as pennyroyal, chickweed, anise or senna herb) contaminated with spores. In the absence of these known infection sources, botulism in babies is associated with aerosols dragged along by the wind, containing spores (for example, Mendoza).

HOW TO PREVENT BOTULISM?

Spores are heat resistant but die with a good sterilization process, which is what happens with industrialized canned foods sold at supermarkets. These are safe as they are subjected to microbiologic controls, carried out both by the manufacturer and by the control and labeling departments.

When *C botulinum* grows in foods (always in the absence of oxygen), a powerful neurotoxin is synthesized, which has a paralyzing effect and acts preventing muscular contraction by inhibiting acetylcholine at somatic motor neurons synapses level in myoneural junctions. A neurotoxin dose as low as 0.1 micrograms is capable of producing the disease.

Botulinic neurotoxins are big proteins ranging from 100 thousand to 200 thousand Daltons (Da). Neurotoxin A is the most deadly, but they are all very sensitive to heat. Namely, *if dealing with a food suspected of being contaminated with botulism, toxins are sensitive to heat and any neurotoxin is rendered inactive by boiling the food for ten minutes or maintaining temperature of 80 °C for 30 minutes.*

IMPORTANT: Absolute safety is only obtained through industrial sterilization or by cooking the food before its consumption. Therefore, one of the prevention alternatives is not consuming the kind of foods of doubtful origin known as "home preserves" or those that are manufactured at "non-registered" facilities (every packaged food must have its number of FCE (Food Canning Establishment) registration and each food packed in it will count with its NRAP (National Registry of Alimentary Products),which offers us certainty that said food has been subjected to an industrial sterilization process with controlled temperatures and time-cycles and then was microbiologically analyzed by a control organism which certifies its innocuousness.

The same may be said of spices, condiments and medicinal herbs sold at street stalls, that are marketed without its origin labeling, their provenance being unknown as well as their subjection to a sterilization process. It must be remembered that microorganisms are normal ground inhabitants.

Honey or "home-grown herb" infusions should not be given to children under one year old, because even though bacteria may not grow or form the toxin on those foods, it may do it in the intestinal tract of this population, which has not yet established its definitive intestinal bacteria, which will probably compete with the microorganism.

Packaged foods whose containers are dented, with leakages or extreme bulges, should not be bought (bacteria may generate gas, provoking the container's swelling). The integrity of the container must be controlled, paying special attention to its seams, before acquiring it.

WHAT ARE THE SYMPTOMS OF BOTULISM?

After the toxin was consumed, it had a 12- to 36-hour incubation period. An adult patient with botulism characteristically shows:

- "Double" vision or blurred vision.

- Dilated pupils that do not respond to light.
- Dry mouth.
- Limb paralysis with progressive respiratory difficulty.
- Palpebral ptosis or drooping of the upper eyelid.

Patients are lucid and without fever. The symptoms have a swift outcome, but if they survive, recovery takes months.

In infants, botulism is due to spore consumption and toxin production in their digestive tube interior. The clinical manifestation includes:

- Faint crying.
- Weak suction.
- Loss of head support.
- Inexpressive face.
- Constipation.
- Urinary retention.

HOW IS BOTULISM TREATED?

Given the swift ending of this disease, treatment is performed taking into account clinical symptoms, without waiting for the microbiological confirmation. Polyvalent antitoxin Type ABE is administered to adults, as it blocks botulinic neurotoxin; in addition, the patient is treated with gastric lavage, enemas and laxatives.

HOW TO AVOID BOTULIN TOXIN DEVELOPMENT IN FOODS?

- Avoid spore germination in foods, keeping them at a temperature of 4 °C (not at room temperature) or at least within an acidic environment (vinegar, for example). Acidic or very acidic foods do not allow the development of the toxin; however, there exist conditions that alkalinize a food, as when there is fungus growth in a canned food interior, for example in tomato cans.
- Due to their origin, vegetables are usually contaminated by bacteria spores and allow outbreaks when they are preserved in a homemade

way, for example, vacuum-packed cabbage salad or sautéed onions, as they are covered with a margarine layer which brings about an anaerobic environment that is favorable for the toxin development. To prevent botulism, therefore, foods should not be stored in anaerobiosis conditions: special precautions should be taken, among others, with pickled vegetables. Failures in these kinds of preserves are basically associated with inadequate technical knowledge.

- Employing correct fruit and vegetable hygiene, washing them under abundant drinking water, and subsequently submerging them (for ten minutes) in a sodium hypochlorite solution (bleach), using two drops of disinfectant per liter of water.
- Educating those who carry out homemade packaging and other food conservation techniques regarding time, preparation and adequate temperatures required for killing spores and regarding the need for refrigerating non-completely processed foods and the efficacy of boiling home bottled or packed vegetables for ten minutes at a minimum, while they are shaken thoroughly, so as to destroy botulinic toxins.
- Correctly washing kitchen utensils and surfaces in contact with foods, applying detergent and hot water and using hot water and soap for hands after touching raw meat or sea products, before preparing foods and after going to the lavatory.
- The food types involved in cases and outbreaks vary according to conservation and diet habits of different countries. It is important to know that any food that permits the microorganism multiplication and its toxin generation due to an inadequate process that allows the spore survival or that is not heated before its consumption entails a highly probable risk of botulism occurrence.
- Homemade preserves based on meat are not recommended. Any food in which signs of bad conditions or spoiling are observed, whether by gas presence in the package, a spurious smell or any other alteration type, must be rejected.
- Given that honey contains *C botulinum* spores, it is an infection source for infants; children under 12 months of age should not consume honey.
- It is necessary to emphasize that in more than one botulism case, some people have expressed that the contaminated food that they consumed was identical to a normal food. That is why, before it is consumed, all homemade preserves must be heated without exception.

- When they are produced and controlled in a rigorous manner, industrial preserves are not usually a cause of botulism. Notwithstanding this, accidents may occur once the canning sterilization ends and a spore entrance from outside is accidentally facilitated through small cracks in the container, when the food sterilization has been inadequate or if time or temperatures of sterilization are inferior to those that are needed for killing spores. In packaged foods, conservation requirements indicated in the package must be followed. The integrity of the package seams and the absence of pores or fissures must be controlled. Therefore, using a correct manufacturing technology is enough for preventing botulism in industrial preserves. *Clostridium botulinum* survival in industrial processes are due to deficient acidification, deficient heat treatment, and wrong usage of nitrites during the process of curing meat.
- Bacteria may or may not produce convexed packages tops and contents with rancid smell. Other contaminants may cause the same effect in cans or bottles. Foods contained in bulging containers should not be opened, and food with a rancid smell should neither be consumed nor "tasted."
- Confitures, jams, marmalades, compotes and fruits preserved in syrup, fruit purée or paste can be manufactured with fruit. In these kind of preserves, the addition of sugar in equal parts to the fruit employed (per fruit kg, a kg of sugar), which is typical of the fruit elaboration process, makes the development of botulism impossible.
- It is important to state that sweeteners do not exert the same preservative effect as that of sugar and as they are placed in considerable lesser proportions, they are not as effective for conservation means and therefore much more severe thermal treatment is required to that effect.
- The most frequent cause of food botulism is the homemade production and consumption of preserves, which are processed in an inappropriate manner, creating an anaerobic environment that encourages spore survival, its germination, reproduction and toxin synthesis.

In short: botulism has often been produced by homemade foods in closed containers and with slightly acidic contents, such as asparagus, green beans, sugar beets and corn. However, epidemic botulism outbreaks have resulted from more unusual sources such as garlic preserved in oil, tomatoes, carrot juice, oven baked potatoes incorrectly handled when wrapped in aluminum paper, meat preserves and homemade preserved fish or fermented and consumed food without correct cooking.

- In the great majority of cases, a safe homemade preserve has an annual duration if and when containers are kept closed and stored in adequate conditions (dry and dark place, cool, under 25-30 °C) and without stacking containers. Once opened, a container must be kept in the refrigerator and be preferably consumed within the space of a week, having previously been heated to destroy the neurotoxin.
- People who prepare homemade preserves should follow the procedures described for reducing food contamination. Garlic-or herb-flavored oils must be refrigerated. Potatoes that have been oven cooked and wrapped in aluminum paper must be kept warm until they are served, within two hours of their preparation, or otherwise be kept in the refrigerator.
- Given that the botulinic toxin is destroyed at high temperatures, those who are going to consume home-stored products should boil foods for ten minutes to ascertain said products are safe for consumption.

A botulism episode occurrence does not confer immunity towards subsequent episodes.

REFERENCES

Rebagliati, V; Chianelli, S; Tornese, M; Rossi, ML; Troncoso, A. Documented outbreak of botulism: the impact of food-borne transmission. *Asian Pac. J. Trop. Med.* 2008; 1 (2): 71-75.

Rebagliati, R; Tornese, M; Troncoso, A. Food-borne botulism in Argentina. *J. Infect. Dev. Ctries.* 2009; 3(4):250-254.

Troncoso, A; Garcia-Moreno, I. The danger of underestimating the risks related to the consumption of contaminated food, Buenos Aires, Cuentahilos eds, 2011.

Troncoso, A; Ruthanne, C. Outbreak Foodborne disease, Buenos Aires, Socrate eds, 2012.

Troncoso, A ; Baron AP. Toxi-Infection Alimentaire-Risques sanitaires liés à l'eau et à l'alimentation.Le livre que vous ne pouvez pas vous premettre d'ignorer, Buenos Aires, Socrate eds, 2012.

Chapter 2

ESCHERICHIA COLI AND HEMOLYTIC-UREMIC SYNDROME (HUS)

HUS in Argentina has an annual incidence that triples that of the rest of countries, with more than 17 cases per 100,000 children under five years old, and around 400 of the new cases that appear each year surpass the totality of cases occurring in the rest of the world. This endemic disease constitutes the first cause of acute renal insufficiency in children younger than five years old, the second cause of chronic renal insufficiency and is responsible for 20% of renal transplant in children and adolescents, as we will see below.

WHAT IS HUS?

HUS is an alimentary infection that causes anemia, decrease of blood platelets and renal failure. It is produced by the enterohemorragic *Escherichia coli* (EHEC) bacteria. Although its presentation varies, a classic symptom is blood in diarrhea, but diarrhea can also be watery. Unlike other infections, the absence of fever is what usually characterizes *E coli* infection. EHEC does not form spores, and that is why it is eliminated during the pasteurization/cooking processes. It grows in a wide range of temperatures (2.5°C-44.5°C), and the optimum temperature is near 37°C; it is resistant to pHs that are acid, and it may grow with or without oxygen.

HUS complications specifically appear in kidneys, with the possibility of developing permanent lesions that will be equivalent to a chronic renal failure. It can also affect the brain; causing then convulsive crisis that may ultimately provoke a coma and permanent consequences that will condition a lifelong cognitive disability. Total recuperation ranges approximately between 60-70% of the affected patients, and relapses are seldom. Around 5% of those who survive carry renal or neurological consequences.

HOW IS HUS TRANSMITTED?

Its main transmission route is minced meat and beef hamburgers. The main *E coli* natural reservoir is cattle, which lodges it in its intestinal tract. It is estimated that more than two-thirds of calves and healthy cows are intestinal carriers of some *E coli* type. Although the number of bacteria required for causing the disease is unknown, it is suspected of being a small quantity.

Meat is contaminated during the animal's slaughter, and microorganisms can fully mix with meat when it is minced. Infected meat is similar to that not infected, as its taste, smell and color are not modified. Contamination may have its origin in a single animal, but meat may be mixed with that of other healthy animals during its processing. Contaminated meat may protect bacteria inside the product when it is used for manufacturing sausages or hamburgers (foods that are often identified as vehicles); therefore bad cooking may let out free a viable microorganism inoculants.

The bacteria responsible for HUS has also been isolated in the digestive tubes and stools of several domestic and wild animals, amongst which are sheep, horses, pigs, turkey, dogs, seagulls and rats. Foods directly or indirectly related to animals (meat or dairy products) as those of animal waste (bovine manure is an important source of infections) have been identified as bacteria transmission vehicles. The presence of microorganisms in stools generates re-infection in cattle and the environment's contamination.

Depending on environmental conditions, *E coli* may survive in cattle stools for 40 to 70 days. If the ground is fertilized with contaminated manure, vegetable consumption would facilitate bacteria transmission. It is also transmitted through drinking, swimming or playing in contaminated waters, and by direct contact (stroking or kissing) with infected animals in farms or zoos.

HOW IS HUS PREVENTED?

Although badly cooked minced meat is the main transmission route, it is not the only way of becoming infected, hence, our responsibility is to generate prevention actions, as children and adolescent's health is at stake. *E coli* is easily passed on from one person to another; therefore it is necessary to take precautions. Inadequate hand hygiene favors secondary spreading through interpersonal contact. Small children who are not toilet-trained are efficient bacteria spreaders. As a result, family members and such children's playmates are subjected to a high risk of becoming infected. It must be remembered that, after intestinal evacuation, washing hands with soap is still the main prevention measure for infections transmitted through stool contamination of the foods that later will be consumed.

HYGIENE

Wash hands well with water and liquid soap:

- Before eating or handling foods,
- After going to the lavatory,
- After touching raw foods,
- After changing diapers,
- After touching animals,
- Before touching cooked or ready to be consumed foods.

FOOD HANDLING

- Cook meats very well (both minced and whole pieces); they must have inside a grayish color but never pink. The adequate cooking of foods destroys microorganisms. They can be boiled, roasted, braised, sautéed, steam cooked, grilled, oven roasted or microwaved, making sure that they are subjected to a temperature of 80 °C.
- Reheating, as well as cooking, should be done at a minimum of 80 °C. It is advisable to perform it in one step and to discard what has not been consumed. When the microwave oven is used for reheating or

cooking food, it must be ensured that no "cold points" remain, as this system heats foods in an uneven way.

- When foods are prepared, do not use the same utensils (knives, kitchen counters, tables) with which raw meat has been cut for another food preparation, especially vegetables or other ingredients that will not be cooked.

Did you know that you should not use the same chopping board for cutting meat and vegetables?

- Avoid contact of meat with other foods, as well as contact of ready foods with raw ones.
- Fruits and vegetables should be always washed carefully under plenty of running, drinkable water. Green leafy vegetables that are employed raw should be washed leaf by leaf—not just the whole plant—first performing a previous rinse of each leaf under running water for discarding visible dirt and then submerging the leaves (for ten minutes) in a bleach solution, in a proportion of two bleach drops per each liter of water (it can be measured with a dropper).
- All dairy products, as well as fruit juices or ciders, must be pasteurized and well kept in cold storage or vacuum packed.
- Avoid consuming products that are manufactured in premises not approved by sanitary authorities or sold at street stalls.
- With respect to food transportation, it is of utmost importance to strictly respect the cold chain for their correct conservation until consumption.

Storage is another important stage: refrigerator's temperature must be kept below 5 °C, in addition to controlling its hygiene and the order of food to be kept inside, placing foods in such a way that cross contamination is avoided: that is, cooked foods, clean vegetables and all food that is ready to be consumed must always be placed higher than raw foods.

WATER

- Water used and meant for consumption should be drinkable water. If its origin is not sure, it should be boiled. When in the street or in restaurants, consume bottled water coming from known brands.

- Avoid immersion in public or home swimming-pools lacking chlorinated water.

When in the countryside, zoos or places where people are in contact with farm animals or with surfaces which they frequent:

- Establish one-way circulation paths.
- Minimize direct contact with animals (kisses, strokes, bottle-feeding, hugs).
- Have a trained staff able to control risks and alert visitors.
- Provide installations for hand-washing nearby the walk circuits exit.
- Install areas where food is served far away from the zone where animals are kept and also install there places adequately equipped for washing hands.
- Avoid marketing sticky foods within the facilities, and if this is not possible, only sell them in "clean" areas.
- Provide brochures and set up posters or billboards for informing about possible dangers and how to proceed inside the premises to avoid infections.
- Inform visitors that calves are animals not suitable for being treated as pets.
- Recommend that sweet and sticky food (lollipops, cotton candies) should only be sold and consumed in farms' and zoos' "clean areas," etc. Ideally, its consumption should be discouraged.

WHAT CAN PRIVATE COMPANIES DO FOR PREVENTING AN OUTBREAK APPEARANCE?

Those companies that provide food services to huge population groups (industrial cafeterias, canteens, hospital and others) should define their raw meat material and fruit and vegetables shopping with a hygienic-sanitary evaluation of their suppliers, in such a way that they can begin by agreeing on technical specifications regarding microbiological quality (among others), which will allow them as the company that supplies the services to identify potential risks, in a first phase; and with regard to the potential risks in its suppliers qualifications, to identify as quickly as possible the most promissory candidates. This will help to keep at a minimum scale the risks implied in choosing adequate raw material for the food product to be manufactured, which, after all, will be translated in social benefits (assisted population will consume a product safe from its production process) and economic (as the company will save further costs before the presence of microbiological or other kind of deviations).

Private companies should evaluate their raw material suppliers through hygienic sanitary monitoring, making sure before they decide on the purchase that they have certified quality norms (minimally Good Agricultural Practices and Good Manufacturing Practices) thus ensuring that price is not to be the only quality standard.

ALL GREENS ARE DANGEROUS: SAFETY STARTS AT THE FARM

One must wash fruits and vegetables that cannot be thoroughly peeled, especially if they are not going to be cooked before eating them. Elderly people, with a fragile immunologic system and children under five years old should not eat alfalfa sprouts, nor spinach, lettuce, radishes or cabbage. Therefore, risk groups (comprised of children, adolescents, older adults) must abstain from consuming these foods in their raw states. The risk lies in the fact that once contamination is produced in food through the use in the farm of cattle manure (usually as a fertilizer), it is extremely difficult to decontaminate food and completely eliminate the risk it possesses, in spite of an exhaustive and detailed washing.

In other words, risk groups should not eat lettuce, radishes or fresh spinach (raw) in particular, alone or in mixed salads. On the other hand, it is safe to eat frozen or canned spinach. E $coli$ O157:H7 bacteria can be killed if spinach is cooked for 15 seconds at 90 °C or in boiling water. If spinach is cooked in a frying pan and not all its parts reach a temperature of 90 °C, it is possible that not all bacteria will die.

If consumers decide to cook spinach, they should avoid that raw spinach contaminates other foods and surfaces which are in contact with other foods, and they should wash their hands and wash all cooking utensils and surfaces with hot water and soap before, during the whole process, and after touching spinach. People who present diarrhea after eating lettuce, fresh spinach or mixed salads containing them should immediately visit a physician and ask him to perform a fecal test for the detection of $E.$ $coli$.

RECOMMENDATIONS TO CONSUMERS

People are often infected with *E coli* 0157: H7 by eating badly cooked minced beef meat. Therefore, families should cook all minced meats as well as hamburgers using a meat digital instant-reading thermometer, as minced meat may darken before bacteria-causing diseases are eliminated. Temperature may be checked by inserting a thermometer in several parts of the hamburger, especially in its thicker section. Be sure that at least 90 ºC is read. If you do not use a thermometer, you may diminish the risk of contracting HUS, looking over minced meat to be sure that there is no pink color in its center.

If you are served a badly cooked hamburger or other minced meat products at a restaurant, send them back and ask for a full cooking. Do not forget to also ask for a clean plate. As any kind of minced beef meat can contain germs that cause diseases, the consumer public in general is urged to observe good hygiene habits and alimentary safety measures and to observe the following advice:

REFRIGERATE MEAT VERY WELL

Refrigerate raw meat within two hours after you have bought it. If after cooking meat and poultry they are not consumed, refrigerate them in the first two hours after they are cooked. Defrost raw meat in a microwave oven or the refrigerator. Do not leave meat on the counter after defrosting.

COOK MEAT WELL

Use a thermometer for measuring internal temperature; this is the only way for ensuring that minced beef is cooked at a sufficiently high temperature for killing harmful bacteria.

Color is NOT a reliable indicator for checking that minced beef or beef hamburgers have been cooked at a sufficiently high temperature for killing harmful bacteria such as *E coli* O157:H7.

SIMPLE PRECAUTIONS MAY BE HELPFUL
FOR PREVENTING HUS

- Cook meat very well as a whole piece.
- Keep your kitchen clean.
- To maintain food in good condition, remember that all food should be processed and cleaned, and separate what is raw from what is cooked, then cook and refrigerate.
- Drink only pasteurized milk, juice or cider.
- Wash fruits and vegetables.
- Drink only drinkable water.
- Wash hands with liquid soap.

In restaurants, even well-cooked foods may be the cause of HUS as they may have been cross contaminated; because of this, risk groups, children in particular, should abstain from eating outside their homes.

Home-prepared hamburgers with minced meat bought at a butcher's shop or supermarket are also risky; they should not be consumed.

Hamburgers industrially manufactured are made with mixtures of minced meat, and nothing ensures that they do not contain the bacteria or its dangerous toxin; they are not appropriate food for children.

Risks of meat minced outside home are applicable to any food that may contain it, for example turnovers (*empanadas*) among others, which for that reason are banned for vulnerable groups.

Keppe, also known according to the zone as *kebbe* or *kepi*, is an Arab food. It is a sort of meatball that can be made with beef as well as with lamb and is usually eaten raw; these are banned for vulnerable groups.

The only safe hamburgers are those that are prepared at home, starting from a whole piece of meat and using the domestic meat mincer.

Yoghurt of industrial origin may also contain bacteria, as it is possible that during its freight or at its selling point the cold chain may have been lost; it is banned for vulnerable groups.

For eliminating bacteria from foods, the most efficacious treatments are cooking, pasteurization and irradiation, provided that, in case of cooking, temperature gets to 80°C at the center of food.

REFERENCES

Rossi, ML; Cricelli, C; Tornese, M; Troncoso, A. Childhood hemolytic syndrome (HUS) in Argentina, epidemiological features and risk factors: when hamburguer becomes a bad word. Viral evolution and its relevance for virus transmission via food. *Pres. Med. Argent.* 2007; 94 (4): 227-237.

Troncoso, A. Hemolytic-uremic syndrome: 25th anniversary of its emergence. Buenos Aires, Stanley editor, 2009.

Watson, D; Escandarani, E; Troncoso, A. Radiation on the dining table. *Rev. Chil. Infectol.* 2009; 26 (4): 318-330.

Troncoso, A.; Bär, N. Food-borne diseases. How to prevent diseases transmitted by food, Buenos Aires, Rene Baron Foundation, 2011.

Troncoso, A; Garcia-Moreno, I. The danger of underestimating the risks related to the consumption of contaminated food, Buenos Aires, Cuentahilos eds, 2011.

Troncoso, A; Ruthanne, C. Outbreak Foodborne disease, Buenos Aires, Socrate eds, 2012.

Troncoso, A ; Baron AP. Toxi-Infection Alimentaire-Risques sanitaires liés à l'eau et à l'alimentation.Le livre que vous ne pouvez pas vous premettre d'ignorer, Buenos Aires, Socrate eds, 2012.

Chapter 3

LISTERIOSIS

Between November 2000 and January 2001, in North Carolina, the United States of America, a listeriosis outbreak was associated with a Mexican-style homemade cheese, made with unpasteurized milk from a local dairy shop.

The affected people were Mexican immigrants. In an initial interview, the great majority of patients revealed that they had eaten an unlabelled Mexican-style mild fresh cheese, bought either in local markets or from a door–to-door selling vendor. There were 11 women in the 12 identified cases with an average age of 21 years old (18-38 years old) and a 70-year-old immuno-compromised man. Ten of the women were pregnant, and the *L monocytogenes* infection led to five dead fetuses, three premature babies and two infected newborn babies. The eleventh woman in her fifth puerperium month showed up at a local hospital with meningitis caused by *L monocytogenes,* without having shown any pre-existing medical condition. All cases were confirmed through laboratory tests.

It was more likely that patients and controlled subjects had consumed any cheese bought from street vendors, Mexican-style fresh cheese and *hot dogs*. Several members of the immigrant Hispanic community elaborated the Mexican-style mild fresh cheese at their homes with raw milk. The inspectors found the Mexican cheese without a label in three of the local Latin shops that they visited in Winston Salem. The owners of two local dairy shops (from Forsyth County) disclosed that they had sold raw milk, from which samples were taken for analysis; there were also samples taken from three neighboring counties dairy shops.

Bacteria was isolated in samples obtained from nine patients, in three cheese samples obtained from stores, in a cheese sample from a patient's home and in a dairy shop raw milk sample. An investigation was performed in a cow farm for determining the bacteria contamination source. Milk samples were obtained from 49 cows and from the storage tank, with no traces of *L monocytogenes*. Therefore, it was concluded that the cows were not infected and that the contamination may have been originated in the environment. As a result of this outbreak, North Carolina sanitary authorities prohibited the selling of raw cow milk in cow farms, educated the store keepers about not selling non-regulated dairy products and recommended reinforcing and increasing the community knowledge about the perils brought by eating, during pregnancy, fresh cheese elaborated with unpasteurized milk.

In this outbreak, it was observed that even though laws may ban the sale and consumption of raw milk and dairy products, as was the case in North Carolina, in some communities, such practices will persist as a result of taste preferences for such cheese types and for cultural reasons. It is regrettable, but the renowned Mexican-style homemade fresh cheese elaborated with unpasteurized milk has caused since the '80s several outbreaks in Hispanic communities, with septic abortions in pregnant women ascribed to *L monocytogenes*. Besides, the fact that in 28 other states raw milk sale to consumers is permitted makes the population's alimentary education difficult, and as the cheese in these communities is produced in private homes, it is difficult to ensure compliance with sanitary regulations. An additional obstacle results from the existing difficulty due to language and other cultural and social barriers for successfully communicating public health messages to the Hispanic community regarding the risk implied in the consumption of this type of product.

The association of listeriosis with milk consumption supports the hypothesis of *Listeria monocytogenes* being a pathogen transmitted to humans through foods deriving from the infected animals or its dairy products. Results suggest that *in sporadic listeriosis, milk should be considered a possible vehicle* and that although pasteurization is a highly effective method for eliminating milk pathogens, it may not be 100% effective.

WHAT IS LISTERIOSIS?

Listeriosis is an infection caused by *L monocytogenes*, a widely distributed pathogenic bacterium that is usually present in the environment; it has been isolated in a variety of sources, including earth, vegetation, mammals and birds' feces, sewages and water. It survives for long periods of time in the environment. The listeriosis bacterium is resistant to several environmental conditions, such as high salinity, which allows it to survive more time under adverse conditions and be able to transmit alimentary diseases. *L monocytogenes* does not form spores, and that is why it is eliminated during the pasteurization/cooking processes. It develops in temperatures near 0°C and 45°C (it grows in a cooling temperature). It grows with or without oxygen. It does not grow with pHs that are acidic (less than 4.5). It is a temporary intestinal resident in 10% of the population, and it is asymptomatic.

It is widely present in places where food is handled, and it can survive for long periods in foods, food processing facilities and private houses, in particular at refrigeration and storage temperatures. It grows in a range of temperatures in between -1.5 and 45 °C.

Foods most frequently associated with human listeriosis are ready-to-be consumed products, which, by definition, are not cooked; in addition, they have a long conservation time period in refrigeration conditions (which does not avoid bacteria reproduction) and are ingested with no treatment for killing the bacteria before they are consumed. For example, these foods include unpasteurized milk, cheeses, butters and other by-products elaborated with said milk, and raw or badly cooked meat, among others. It is also present in vegetal foods and in cooked meals, if contaminated after being processed.

Listeria monocytogenes is a pathogen that when found in foods can cause serious diseases, mainly in high-risk groups such as immuno-compromised people, pregnant women and neonates. It is the first cause of abortions, blood poisoning or infection at the central nervous system level. In the past, outbreaks were linked to a great variety of foods, in particular processed meats (sausages, pâté, pre-cooked products); currently, the majority of cases is connected to consumption of raw milk or cheeses made with unpasteurized milk.

WHAT ARE THE SYMPTOMS OF LISTERIOSIS?

It may cause an asymptomatic infection; manifestation is similar to flu symptoms, gastroenteritis (diarrhea, nausea, and vomiting), meningitis, blood poisoning (widespread infection). It may cause in pregnant women spontaneous abortions and premature childbirth, newborn baby with meningitis or sepsis, and death of the baby.

WHO IS AT RISK?

- Children.
- Old-age people (more than 50 years old).
- Pregnant women and their fetuses.
- Immunosuppressed (transplanted patients in corticoid chronic treatment).

HOW IS LISTERIOSIS PREVENTED?

As this microorganism is widely distributed throughout nature, the approach both at consumer level and in the alimentary industry should not be focalized in preventing its presence but, rather, in minimizing its levels in foods. Then:

WHICH PREVENTION MEASURES WE CAN ADOPT AS CONSUMERS?

- Avoid consuming unpasteurized milk, soft cheeses, blue-veined cheeses (Roquefort, Camembert) and any other food that has been elaborated with "raw milk."
- Consume cheese manufactured at industrial level, with an intact original packaging and a label indicating pasteurized milk among its ingredients.
- To cook food at more than 80 °C is an effective measure, as bacteria do not resist such temperatures.
- Consume foods at a temperature higher than 72 °C and within two hours of being prepared.
- Reheat ready–to-consume foods at more than 80 °C.
- Do not perform defrosting of meat products at room temperature; the correct procedure is from freezer to refrigerator and from refrigerator to cooking.
- Pregnant women should consume boiled pasteurized milk, sterilized milk, hard cheeses and yogurt manufactured with pasteurized milk.
- Keep cooked foods in the refrigerator in a separate compartment from cheeses and from raw foods.

- Do not let raw foods juices drip into other foods during its storage; that's why the norm that establishes that "all that is cooked and ready for consumption should always be placed above what is raw" must be followed.
- Do not handle raw foods with the same elements used for cooked foods. First, utensils must be washed in a hot water and detergent solution and correctly rinsed (without leaving soap traces). Utensils should never be washed only with water.
- In first place, adequately wash vegetables and fruits under running water and afterwards submerge them in a water and chlorine solution (two drops per liter of utilized water).
- Avoid consuming raw or badly cooked, salted or smoked beef, chicken and fish (also avoid pink juices).
- Consume perishable foods and/or ready-to-be consumed foods as soon as possible after buying them.
- Wash hands with water and soap after handling raw foods.
- Regularly clean the refrigerator with water and neutral soap and disinfect it with a sodium hypochlorite solution in water, observing the dose indicated by the manufacturer.

BANNED FOOD FOR RISK GROUPS

1) Do not consume processed meats or sausage *chacinados* products unless they are piping hot and steaming.
2) Avoid fluid in sausage packages coming into contact with other foods, utensils and food preparation counters. Be sure of washing hands after coming into contact with any kind of cold cut or processed meat.
3) Do not consume Feta, Brie and Camembert type mild cheeses; such as blue cheese, Roquefort; or Mexican style white cheese, fresh cheese, and Panela cheese; unless in the label it is clearly stated that they are manufactured with pasteurized milk.
4) Do not consume homemade pâtés with spreading consistency or meat pastes, such as mortadella type. They can be consumed in its canned presentation as they have been sterilized.
5) Do not consume refrigerated smoked shellfish, unless they are cooked.

6) Do not consume refrigerated smoked marine products, unless they are part of a dish that requires its cooking. Canned shellfish varieties may be consumed.

7) Do not consume hot dogs or cooked sliced meat, unless they are reheated with hot steam.

8) Selected foods known as delicatessen (*Delikatessen*) are risky and include, among others, pickled dishes (*escabeches*), smoked foods, salted tuna filets, caviar, artichokes, beans, anchovies, asparagus, Aguinaga Eels, Bomba de Calasparra Rice, Esla Valleys Meats, Priest's Orchard Dates (Elche), Denia Red Shrimp, Fuentesáuco Chickpeas, Raf Tomatoes. A product qualifies as a delicatessen when it keeps the region's spirit and its handcrafted nature, without losing its presence and quality when exhibited or tasted by an attentive palate, notwithstanding the risks associated with its "exquisiteness." An innocuous food is indistinguishable from a contaminated one either by its taste, aroma, texture or aspect.

9) Abstain from acquiring products in "delis." A "deli" is a restaurant that also has direct-sale products for the general public. Travelers should take this into account, for instance, if they want to know the authentic New York food. Maybe the two best known "delis" in New York include Katz, on Houston Street, in the middle of Lower East Side, one of Manhattan neighborhoods. The other best known "deli" is Cargenie's Delicattesen on the Seventh Avenue, very close to Times Square. However, if you belong to a risk group and are invited to taste an authentic New York dish, as for example, an enormous Hot Pastrami Sandwich, you better not to try it!

MEASURES THAT THE ALIMENTARY INDUSTRY SHOULD ADOPT FOR OFFERING A SAFE PRODUCT

- Food industry may minimize risks by implementing quality norms to systematize the cleaning and disinfection of utilized equipment and utensils, including, for example, Sanitation Standard Operative Procedures (SSOP), which describes the sanitation tasks applied before (pre-operational) and during elaboration (operational) processes.

SSOP should clearly state steps to be followed for ensuring compliance with cleaning and disinfection requirements. It should be stated in a clear manner how these steps should be performed, with what elements, when, and by whom. For achieving its purposes, they must be totally explicit, clear and detailed, avoiding any distortion or misinterpretation that may cause damage to consumers.

- Ensure food manipulators adequately comply with procedures for obtaining their health files before being employed.

In addition, it must be stressed that listeriosis is a disease created by man, namely, it is a civilization's disease. Its importance for public health has not always been recognized, mainly because when comparing it with other more common diseases as for example salmonellosis, listeriosis is relatively rare. However, due to its high mortality rate, listeriosis is placed among the most frequent causes of death through food-transmitted diseases (it is placed second), after salmonellosis. Changes occurring in food production, storage and distribution have propitiated several outbreaks. In the last decades, many countries have made intense efforts towards listeriosis prevention; the remarkable reduction of its incidence during the nineties suggests a positive relation with implemented measures.

Summing up, *Listeria monocytogenes* is a pathogenic microorganism that, only in the United States, causes 500 deaths every year, most of which could be avoided through the corresponding control in production points. An additional peril appears as *Listeria* can reproduce itself at low temperatures; therefore refrigeration at more than 6 °C is not a safe method against it, for which reason, the European Directive now requires that manufacturers perform controls for its detection, especially in the alimentary industry.

As an example of listeriosis relevance with regard to public health, in November 2006, 17 people had to be hospitalized in the Czech Republic suffering from a serious infection due to *L. monocytogenes*. Three adults and a baby died because of the infection. Thirty people were hospitalized in that country with similar symptoms during the three previous months. All indicates that those patients were ill after having consumed some processed meats or some unpasteurized dairy products.

"We have stopped being sufficiently cautious in the control of some foods. We are careless regarding the detection in foods of the dangerous

Listeria type bacteria," admitted Michael Vít, Health Minister of the Czech Republic.

Once again, this underlines the fact that food microbiological perils characterization should be increased to cover all the components of the host-food-pathogenic agent triangle. The idea of an infection threshold for microbial risks should be rejected, as the present burden of evidence points out that every ingested microorganism has a certain probability (as remote as it may be) of causing disease.

PREVENTIVE MEASURES THAT SHOULD NOT BE FORGOTTEN

- Avoid cross contamination: avoid fluids dripping from the upper part of the fridge and avoid using the same chopping board where you cut the chicken for chopping the tomatoes.
- Correctly defrost foods: put them directly on the fire, in the fridge or in the microwave.
- Consume perishable food or food that is ready to be consumed as soon as possible after it is bought: for example, cold meat that is covered with a Saran wrap, and do not use the same cutter for those that are raw and those that are cured.
- Do not consume sausages or cold meats unless they are hot and steaming.
- Do not consume dairy products that do not have in the label the explanation that such product was obtained from pasteurized milk.
- Do not consume homemade pâté or meat pastes that are not in cans (sterilization process). For example: Leberwurst.
- Do not consume smoked marine products that are refrigerated without cooking before the consumption. *You can consume them when they are canned.*
- Hot dogs: consume them only at home, after the sausages have been cooked (boil them for three minutes) or choose the ones that are pasteurized.
- Avoid that the sausage fluids get in contact with other food, cooking utensils and surfaces where the food is prepared.

- Make sure that the personnel have good hygienic practices, such as washing their hands, and ensure that there is extreme hygiene in the slabbing and packaging areas.
- Establish areas that are properly separated in order to completely separate the cooked products from the raw ones.

To Take into Account

Listeria monocytogenes is more lethal than other pathogenic agents that are more well known, such as *Salmonella* and *E coli*, although, in general, epidemics with these germs cause more sick people than dead people.

References

Rossi, ML; Paiva, A; Tornese, M; Chianelli, S; Troncoso, A. *Listeria monocytogenes* outbreaks: a review of the routes that favor bacterial presence. *Rev. Chil. Infectol.* 2008; 25 (5): 328-335.

Tornese, M; Paiva, A; Watson, D; Chianelli, S; Rossi ML; Troncoso A. *Listeria monocytogenes* and human listeriosis, a food borne pathogen: review of the literature. *Pres. Med. Argent.* 2008; 95 (1): 26-34.

Rebagliati, V; Philippi, R; Rossi ML; Troncoso A. Prevention of foodborne listeriosis. *Indian J. Pathol. Microbiol.* 2009;52 (2):145-149.

Troncoso, A.; Bär, N. Food-borne diseases. How to prevent diseases transmitted by food, Buenos Aires, Rene Baron Foundation, 2011.

Troncoso, A; Garcia-Moreno, I. The danger of underestimating the risks related to the consumption of contaminated food, Buenos Aires, Cuentahilos eds, 2011.

Troncoso, A; Ruthanne, C. Outbreak Foodborne disease, Buenos Aires, Socrate eds, 2012.

Troncoso, A ; Baron AP. Toxi-Infection Alimentaire-Risques sanitaires liés à l'eau et à l'alimentation.Le livre que vous ne pouvez pas vous premettre d'ignorer, Buenos Aires, Socrate eds, 2012.

Chapter 4

HEPATITIS A

In 2004, there was an important outbreak of hepatitis A in Egypt, in which 351 patients from nine European countries were involved. For approximately 6 to 21 days, all patients were guests at the same hotel. Of a total of 351 cases, there were 271 primary cases in Germany and seven secondary cases, besides 60 informed primary cases in other eight European countries. Austria recorded a secondary outbreak with 13 cases, which were caused by an infected food handler who had been lodged at said hotel. The outbreak was originated by the consumption of orange juice served at the breakfast buffet, which had been probably contaminated during its elaboration process, whether by an infected worker with inadequate hand hygiene or by contact with sewage waste that contaminated fruit or machinery. It was observed that the risk of contracting hepatitis A was significantly increased by high doses of juice. The fact that juice was consumed by 60% of healthy control cases may be explained in part by the fluctuation of virus concentration within the juice, which resulted in different infectiousness degrees. The risk of contracting hepatitis A significantly increased with higher juice doses.

Tourists were telephone interviewed to determine, among other things, which foods and beverages they had consumed, and if they had taken part during their stay in recreational activities. The study included people whose positive clinical analysis indicated they had been infected by the virus, as well as people with no laboratory evidence of the disease who had also traveled with them. Vaccination of the hotel guests and of their employees was one of the preventive measures implemented by the hotel.

Sandwiches, salads and fresh fruit prepared by infected food handlers have also been implied in hepatitis A outbreaks. A great number of people may be at risk, if food is centrally prepared by restaurants and then is widely distributed to different meeting points.

A United States outbreak involved a catering company that employed a food handler infected with hepatitis A; 91 hepatitis A cases were subsequently identified through 21 of the 41 events that that company serviced.

In another outbreak, 230 people were infected by an employee who worked in two sandwich elaboration premises. Two similar outbreaks occurred among people who ate bakery products contaminated by feces of a handler excreting hepatitis A, then contaminating the sugar glaze applied to baked products.

In the United Kingdom, more than 50 residents of a village group were infected after eating either unwrapped bread, rolls or snacks offered in a shop whose owner had been ill with hepatitis A. It was concluded that bread had been contaminated by the owner of the shop, whose hands had been inadequately cleaned and presented visible lesions.

Glasses have also been involved in the infection transmission to consumers. In Thailand, an outbreak occurred among college students who had filled their glasses through immersion in a water storage tank at the school cafeteria; the hypothesis is that someone with fecal matter on his hands had contaminated water with the virus. In another outbreak, associated with a United Kingdom public building, infection was ascribed to an infected barman who had probably contaminated the glasses with his hands dirtied with fecal matter.

Since 1940, hepatitis A is known as a disease that propagates by the fecal-oral route, through consumption of foods contaminated by infected food handlers or infected human feces. A group of mollusks known as bivalves (oysters, mussels, cockles, etc.), which are consumed without a prior cooking process, participate in the primary contamination, as they represent the main vehicles of alimentary origin viral diseases. Meats, dairy products, fruits and vegetables are also associated with hepatitis A.

WHAT IS HEPATITIS A?

Hepatitis A is an acutely infectious liver disease caused by a virus. There are 10,000,000 worldwide new cases per year. It is transmitted through consumption of foods or water contaminated by infected human feces or from person to person when hygiene is inadequate and foods are handled.

WHAT ARE THE SYMPTOMS?

- Weakness: very important physical asthenia.
- Jaundice (eyes and skin with a yellow color).
- Nausea.
- Lack of appetite.
- Urine with tea or cola-flavored drink color.
- Putty colored faeces, whitish.

Infection may be asymptomatic, mild, moderate, complicated with prolonged jaundice, yearlong recurrent episodes, or devastating and fatal.

HOW HEPATITIS A IS PREVENTED?

Four verbs are applied in hepatitis A prevention:

- Boil (water if it is not drinkable),
- Cook (hot and steaming foods are safe),
- Peel (raw fruits and vegetables),
- Forget (if it is not possible to gain access to previously stated measures).

"BOIL IT, COOK IT, PEEL IT OR FORGET IT"

Other measures for preventing hepatitis A:

- Adequate elimination of human feces, i.e., through main drainage.
- Drinkable water access.
- Correct hand washing after using the lavatory and before, during and after preparing foods. This means using running drinkable water, soap and nailbrush. Never wash hands only with water.
- Do not drink water and drinks at street stalls or share drinks from spouts, *bombillas* (tube through which mate tea is drunk), nor glasses.
- Avoid consumption of ice when it is not prepared at home, as the origin of the water with which it has been made is unknown.

- It does not reproduce in food, but it survives in raw vegetables which are fecally contaminated and in ice. Adequate fruit and vegetable washing. Many times, during production, fruits and vegetables are watered using contaminated waters or fertilized with products that can function as a primary source of contamination for these foods and transmit the disease when raw salads are consumed. Hence, the importance of washing them under running drinkable water and subsequently submerging them for ten minutes in water with chlorine, using 2 chlorine drops per liter of water proportion.
- Correct food cooking (the safest way is for them to be piping hot and steaming).
- Do not consume raw fish or shellfish; if the latter derive from contaminated waters, they may carry the virus during food filtration process. Virus does not infect these species, but it is lodged for days or weeks in the shellfish digestive system. Unlike many other edible marine products, shellfish are eaten raw or lightly cooked without removing the digestive system. Frequently, it is customary to consume these foods in a raw or insufficiently cooked manner. Raw or insufficiently cooked fish and shellfish may be the cause of a case of hepatitis A.
- Avoid consuming cold foods that require much handling during preparation (such as fruit or vegetable salads, sandwiches, etc.).
- Repeated use of alcohol gel outside home.
- Do not swim in contaminated waters.

In public or private institutions (schools, hospital, factories, restaurants and others):

- Periodically clean drinkable and kitchen employed water tanks and cisterns, with water and chlorine, and record in writing the date when it was carried out.
- In schools, lavatories should be cleaned after each recess with a solution made up with a known brand of sodium hypochlorite in 5 liters of water for five minutes for floors, walls and bathroom fittings. Firstly, water closets should be cleaned with water and detergent solution, totally rinsed and a cup of chlorine should be poured next, brushing well and leaving it to act for five minutes, and lastly, discharge.
- In large cities, where people use public transport and contact with a variety of elements is frequent, it is essential to wash hands when arriving home, and use gel alcohol during transportation.

- Food handlers who present hepatitis A or other diseases should immediately notify their employers and stop working, the latter being responsible for keeping employee(s) from returning to their habitual employment until causes that motivated such separation disappear.
- Adequate hand washing is a crucial point in handlers of large food volumes as they often have the bad habit of only "rinsing" their hands with water, and then drying them, and putting on their disposable gloves and start touching utensils, raw foods, garbage cans, cooked foods, cold chambers door handles, cleaning products, etc., thinking that they are exempted from hand washing by wearing gloves. It must be taken into account that gloves are hands' prolongation and that they should be changed as many times as necessary.

VACCINATION IS THE BEST PREVENTION AGAINST HAV INFECTION

Dead virus vaccine is very safe; it is the most efficient manner of preventing the disease and grants life immunity when patient is correctly immunized with two doses.

TO THINK OVER

Hepatitis A virus can remain alive for several hours on a person's hands and is transferred easily from the hands of an infected food handler onto the food being handled. In the early 1990s, researchers in Ottawa, Canada studied the survival of hepatitis A virus on five volunteers applying a fecal suspension containing a measured quantity of hepatitis A virus on the tips of their fingers and found that up to 30% of the virus could still be detected after four hours, and even after drying for four hours on a volunteer's hands, those living virus particles could still be transferred from the finger tips of the volunteer's hand to metal disks by simple pressure. The researchers also had the volunteers test the effectiveness of several hand-washing products—regular hand soap and germicidal soap—at removing or killing hepatitis A virus. They concluded that most of the products were inadequate; live virus particles could still be transferred to metal disks even after the volunteers washed their hands with common soap or with many of the medical products. Only the use of hand cleaners containing high alcohol levels prevented the transfer of live hepatitis

A particles. In view of how difficult it can be to wash away or kill the virus, free vaccination of food service workers has been proposed as the only way to prevent outbreaks.

NEXT PREVENTION LEVEL IS PERSONAL HYGIENE

Adequate hand washing and the application of correct food handling practices, in particular regarding raw products, stand out. These measures should not be exclusively applied in the alimentary industry. Consumers in general need to have an adequate involvement, as in private homes is where spreading mostly occurs. Thus, if hygienic measures application does not extend in the private sphere, it will proliferate from said sphere toward other places, including from person to person, which will make infeasible the application of other preventive measures.

REFERENCES

Fino, G; Cricelli, C; Rossi, ML; Troncoso, A. Viral evolution and its relevance for virus transmission via food. *Pres Med Argent,* 2008; 95 (3): 559-577.

Troncoso, A; Miranda, A; Paiva, A; Rossi, ML; Puchulu, B. Survival and transport of human enteric viruses in foods. *Pres. Med. Argent.* 2008; 95 (2): 481-499.

Troncoso, A.; Bär, N. Food-borne diseases. How to prevent diseases transmitted by food, Buenos Aires, Rene Baron Foundation, 2011.

Troncoso, A; Garcia-Moreno, I. The danger of underestimating the risks related to the consumption of contaminated food, Buenos Aires, Cuentahilos eds, 2011.

Troncoso, A; Dawson, J. Texbook of Human Virology, Buenos Aires, Socrate eds, 2011.

Troncoso, A; Ruthanne, C. Outbreak Foodborne disease, Buenos Aires, Socrate eds, 2012.

Troncoso, A; Desenclos, MF. Maladies Infectieuses et immunisation, Buenos Aires, Socrate eds, 2012.

Troncoso, A ; Baron AP. Toxi-Infection Alimentaire-Risques sanitaires liés à l'eau et à l'alimentation.Le livre que vous ne pouvez pas vous premettre d'ignorer, Buenos Aires, Socrate eds, 2012.

Chapter 5

HEPATITIS E (HEV)

In 1955, at least 29,000 residents of New Delhi, India, were victims of a Hepatitis E outbreak after drinking fecally contaminated water. This was the first confirmed outbreak of hepatitis E but many would follow. In 1986, in Xinjiang, China, a great outbreak that affected 120,000 people in 23 cities and persisted for 20 months occurred through consumption of fecally contaminated water.

Between May 22 and July 30, 2004, in clinics of the Great Darfur region, Sudan, 625 cases and 22 deaths caused by hepatitis E were reported. Although suspected hepatitis E cases had been reported in East, West and North Darfur, the highest incidence was registered at Morni camp for internally displaced persons, in West Darfur. An analysis of the camp epidemiologic data revealed that 149 cases and eight deaths had been reported. Seventy percent of the cases involved women, and the average age was 24 years old. Of the eight reported deaths, six (75%) corresponded to pregnant women. In fact, as this outbreak documents, HEV (Hepatitis E Virus) may be fatal in up to 20-30% of pregnant women and is particularly dangerous in the third quarter of pregnancy (HEV is fatal in one of five pregnant women).

Another outbreak recorded in Sudan between June 26 and August 13, 2004, was reported by a joint WHO and Sudan Health Ministry collaboration team, where a total of 672 HEV cases and 21 deaths linked to it were reported in Goz Amer, a Sudanese refugee camp. Hepatitis E antibodies' presence in blood samples was confirmed by Val de Grâce, a laboratory in Paris. Both Sudan outbreaks were related to non-drinkable salty water and a sanitary deficit that refugee and internally displaced camps at both sides of Chad and Sudan frontiers suffer.

The research of the risk factors linked with Sudan outbreaks showed that water chlorination was insufficient for deactivating the infectious agent and controlling the epidemic. Chad is one of the ten poorest countries of the world, and its eastern regions are among the most depressed, with very hard agricultural conditions, scarce drinkable water supply, few schools and difficult access to health facilities.

WHAT IS HEPATITIS E?

Enterically transmitted hepatitis E virus is widely spread in many tropical and sub-tropical countries. HEV has multiple transmission routes, by water or fecally contaminated foods, person to person, through raw or badly cooked shellfish or by badly cooked pork meat, swine or domestic pigs are considered a reservoir for HEV.

Traditionally, hepatitis E has been considered, together with hepatitis A, an infectious hepatitis transmitted through the fecal-hydric route. With this epidemiologic pattern, it is recognized in poor countries, where it can cause epidemics, sometimes very important, related with the consumption of contaminated water. Hepatitis E is a viral disease that contributes to identify the status of underdevelopment and of deplorable hygienic conditions in the absence of drinkable water and sewage. HEV causes infections that occur in the form of epidemic outbreaks, as well as isolated sporadic disease cases in many parts of the world.

HOW IS HEPATITIS E TRANSMITTED?

The virus responsible for hepatitis E has multiple transmission routes: water or fecally contaminated foods and raw or badly cooked shellfish. Cases that occurred in Japan—as one involving a family who had consumed raw deer meat three weeks before the appearance of a devastating outbreak—indicate that the virus could also be transmitted through raw or badly cooked pork, wild boar or deer meat or liver.

WHAT ARE HEPATITIS E SYMPTOMS?

Hepatitis E's incubation period is longer than hepatitis A's incubation period. Its duration ranges from 22 to 60 days, with a greater than 40 media. There are asymptomatic as well as symptomatic cases. Clinical manifestations of hepatitis E are identical to those of hepatitis A.

Boiling water before drinking has always been associated with the reduction of the risk of developing this disease. Inadequate handling of excreta is an important contributing factor in the appearance of HEV outbreaks, as human fecally contaminated drinkable water storage areas (reservoir, wells, etc.) facilitate the appearance of this hepatitis virus, i.e., outbreaks are recognized during rainy seasons in deprived health areas, as feces contaminate water storage tanks.

The best way to prevent hepatitis E virus infection is to establish protection mechanisms against fecal contamination in water systems. An adequate handling (purification) of water provided to the population will contribute to avoid infection by this virus. Prevention depends on the protection of provided water and an adequate handling of contaminated waters.

HOW IS HEPATITIS E PREVENTED?

- Hepatitis E is prevented with the same measures previously described for hepatitis A.

Unlike what happens with hepatitis A, there is no vaccine for hepatitis E.
Whichever may be the difficulties, work must go on—both for providing drinkable water, food, and medical assistance and for educating a population that usually is fighting to survive in conditions that in far too many cases, can be described as less than human.

WHO ARE THOSE AT RISK?

- Hepatitis E is particularly dangerous for pregnant women. It may appear in a sudden, devastating manner, and in 30% of gestating mothers who acquire it, it is fatal.

- Those that live exposed to poverty and inadequate health conditions.
- International travelers to developing countries that do not take precautionary measures.
- People with no access to drinking water and lavatory fittings.
- People who consume insufficiently cooked pork or wild boar meat.

REFERENCES

Paiva, A; Rebagliati, V; Troncoso, A. Zoonotic transmission of hepatitis E: implications for public health worldwide. *Asian Pac J Trop Med* 2009; 2 (4):77-82.

Troncoso, A.; Bär, N. Food-borne diseases. How to prevent diseases transmitted by food, Buenos Aires, Rene Baron Foundation, 2011.

Troncoso, A; Garcia-Moreno, I. The danger of underestimating the risks related to the consumption of contaminated food, Buenos Aires, Cuentahilos eds, 2011.

Troncoso, A; Dawson, J. Texbook of Human Virology, Buenos Aires, Socrate eds, 2011.

Troncoso, A; Ruthanne, C. Outbreak Foodborne disease, Buenos Aires, Socrate eds, 2012.

Troncoso, A; Desenclos, MF. Maladies Infectieuses et immunisation, Buenos Aires, Socrate eds, 2012.

Troncoso, A ; Baron AP. Toxi-Infection Alimentaire-Risques sanitaires liés à l'eau et à l'alimentation.Le livre que vous ne pouvez pas vous premettre d'ignorer, Buenos Aires, Socrate eds, 2012.

Chapter 6

TRICHINOSIS

On December 5, 1791, in Vienna, Austria, Wolfgang Amadeus Mozart, bedridden with swelling, pains and vomiting, received the last ministrations of his doctor, Nicolaus Closset. Approximately at midnight, the doctor ordered cold water and vinegar compresses to be put on Mozart's brow, trying to turn down his temperature, but Mozart would die less than one hour later, when he was barely 35 years old. From that moment to now, the death cause of one of the greater geniuses in musical history was subject to innumerable speculations. Among them, trichinosis is pointed out.

WHAT IS TRICHINOSIS?

Trichinosis is caused by *Trichinella spiralis* a microscopic worm hidden in the muscles of pork and other carnivorous animals; 30 grams of sausage or other infected cold cut may contain more than 100,000 infected larvae in cysts. An infected animal may have more than 100,000 worms in larvae stage in all its muscle tissues.

The main hosts of this parasite are rats, pork and human beings. Rats acquire it mainly because of their carnivorous habits, which maintain and propagate the infection in nature. Pigs obtain infection by ingesting infected rats, feeding in garbage heaps, and by ingesting remains of dead animals found at pig farms. An apparently healthy pig does not provide assurance of being parasite free, unlike what is habitually believed. The animal may be in an optimal state for slaughter and then meat veterinary inspection confirms muscular parasitization.

Human beings infect themselves by eating raw or badly or insufficiently cooked pork meat, cold cuts, or homemade *chacinados* or sausages with *Trichinella spiralis* live larvae. On rare occasions, one may be infected through ingestion of other animal-infected meats, such as wild boar, fox, horse, seal or walrus.

WHAT SYMPTOMS DOES TRICHINOSIS PRESENT?

- Fever.
- Upper and lower eyelid edema in both eyes.
- Pink eyes (looks like conjunctivitis).
- Face swelling.
- Severe muscular pains.
- Gastrointestinal symptoms are less frequently present, such as abdominal cramps, nausea and vomiting.

HOW IS TRICHINOSIS PREVENTED?

Prophylactic measures include well-built pigsties, clean, away from garbage dumps and from rats, as well as pig slaughter centralization in facilities subjected to meat inspections carried out by qualified and responsible technical personnel from sanitary control organisms. Veterinarians must examine with a trichinoscope the slaughtered animals' muscle cuts. It is a simple and very low-cost analysis used for enabling a veterinarian and a laboratory to confirm that the animal is infection free. If the pork meat analysis determines trichinosis presence, the meat is not fit for consumption. This control is the only consumer guarantee.

In the Republic of Argentina, SENASA* now employs artificial digestion for visualizing parasites (officially declared method according to Resolution N° 193/96). Said technique enables to increase the sanitary aptitude degree of pork meats fit for consumption, as it presents a greater sensitivity, especially when comparing it with direct trichonoscope technique (Trichonoscope Sensitivity: 3 larvae per gram; digestion sensitivity: 0.1 larvae per gram).

Pigs raised for human food must be correctly fed; it is fundamental to prevent pigs from ingesting garbage or abattoir wastage or restaurant wastes (as there may be waste containing larvae that can infect pigs) and living next to rats, as many times rats are responsible for keeping the disease in a region. Besides, sanitary education should be directed to instill the habit of ingesting adequately cooked pork meat, as it is of vital importance for avoiding trichinosis outbreaks. Homemade sausages are particularly dangerous as they are not controlled by regulatory organisms and are the usual infection cause.

As consumers, we should systematically distrust all "homemade" foods, as not existing at a manufacturing facility, it is not possible to certify that the corresponding controls have been carried out. Avoid buying *chacinados* from street vendors or those offered along the roads. Sausages and cold cuts should only be bought when they present labels on which the following may be checked:

- Product brand
- Responsible company for the elaboration
- Municipal and/or Provincial and/or National authorization of the manufacturing facility
- Elaborating establishment address
- Product elaboration and expiration date
- Product composition
- Conservation temperatures.

If knowledge of the existence of pigsties in bad conditions is obtained, it should be reported to your city municipal authorities. In relation to cooking, meats should be well cooked (be it pork, wild boar, horse or wild animals), never juicy, cooked until its pink color disappears and meat fibers are correctly separated upon cutting (if a meat thermometer is at hand, be sure of more than 80 ºC in the middle of the meat piece). Adequate freezing also eliminates larval cysts (a 15 cm piece of meat at a temperature of –15 ºC for 30 days, or – 25 ºC or less for ten days will destroy them in an effective way in case control barrier was exceeded); but an adequate thermometer must be used.

Salting and smoking DO NOT kill the parasite. It is advisable when having a meal away from home to be sure of the compliance with this procedure, and order a dish that does not include said procedures (it is always better, ideally, to prepare our own food).

REFERENCES

Cricelli, C; Troncoso, A. First case of trichinosis caused by consumption of undercooked horse meat in Argentina. *J. Infect. Dev. Ctries.* 2007; 1(2): 217-219.

Troncoso, A.; Bär, N. Food-borne diseases. How to prevent diseases transmitted by food, Buenos Aires, Rene Baron Foundation, 2011.

Troncoso, A; Garcia-Moreno, I. The danger of underestimating the risks related to the consumption of contaminated food, Buenos Aires, Cuentahilos eds, 2011.

Troncoso, A; Ruthanne, C. Outbreak Foodborne disease, Buenos Aires, Socrate eds, 2012.

Troncoso, A ; Baron AP. Toxi-Infection Alimentaire-Risques sanitaires liés à l'eau et à l'alimentation.Le livre que vous ne pouvez pas vous premettre d'ignorer, Buenos Aires, Socrate eds, 2012.

Chapter 7

BRUCELLOSIS OR MALTA FEVER

Brucellosis was described by Hippocrates in year 450, before Christ. The history of this disease goes back to the island of Malta at the end of the 19th century, where English troops there stationed were attacked by a condition that caused the death of several soldiers. Under these circumstances, in 1904, the English government sent an investigative commission known as the "Mediterranean Fever Commission," presided over by David Bruce, a military anatomopathologist doctor who, as early as 1887, had discovered small microbes in autopsy specimens of increased-in-size spleens obtained from soldiers' deceased at Malta. After one year, he achieved the bacteria isolation and culture that he named *Micrococcus melites.*

Later on, Bruce showed that goats were the infection's main reservoir as he had detected the bacteria in the blood, urine and milk of these animals. This finding paved the way for explaining the disease's epidemiology. For example, as officers drank more milk than soldiers, it was three times more probable that officers were ill with brucellosis. In turn, a great number of cases occurred among hospital interns where milk was amply distributed.

In 1983, an outbreak of brucellosis appeared in Houston, Texas, involving 29 people. It had begun on April 7, when a possible case was reported to the Health Department. Three weeks later, 12 more cases had been recorded and as days went by, cases increased. By July 19, a total of 29 identified cases had been recorded. Patients presented a wide age range, ranging from 2 to 81 years of age. All patients were Mexican immigrants residing in the northeastern section of Houston city. Twenty-eight of the 29 patients reported having eaten goat cheese before symptoms began, and 23 of them had bought it from their car at a local fair. None of the patients who were interviewed had remains of such cheese, but it was possible to purchase an additional piece to perform the corresponding laboratory analysis.

It was proved in the analysis that the cheese came from Linares, Mexico, and that it was not pasteurized. All intents of isolating *Brucella* starting from the cheese failed: however, *Brucellas* were detected in the blood of 20 of the 29 patients. On May 6, the media alerted the population about the potential danger involved in buying cheese from street vendors or street stalls. After such warning, the presence of street vendors was not observed in the town.

This outbreak shows a failure in the United States' customs controls and a failure in the control of street vendors. Although it was only restricted to the Mexican community, the existence of a potential danger for public health was demonstrated. The alert measures performed for preventing cheese consumption were efficient for eliminating the presence of the implied street vendors, but measures to be performed for avoiding the occurrence of other future outbreaks occurring are still missing. It should be noted that conditions of street sales of goat cheese, characterized by lack of hygiene and absence of refrigeration, may have stimulated even more the growth of *Brucella* in goat cheese. Lastly, it can be inferred that cheese storage during its entrance to the United States had been carried out through an inadequately hygienized transport and no refrigeration.

Brucellosis is a disease of great importance in Latin America due to the economic losses it causes to national cattle farming. It affects animal health and productivity, causing infertility, sterility, mastitis and abortions; it reduces approximately 15% of milk production and causes decreases in calves' weight and a diminution in heifer's reproductive efficiency. In addition, brucellosis represents a true occupational risk for people who work directly with animals or with its products, as well as for those who consume unpasteurized milk and its by-products. Even though its real incidence is unknown, it is known that it can be up to 26 times greater than what is officially reported.

WHAT IS BRUCELLOSIS?

Brucellosis is an infectious disease transmitted through animals (or by its products), provoked by a highly virulent bacterium, called *Brucella*. Beef cattle, goats, sheep, and pigs, among others, are the animals that can transmit the disease. These animals may exhibit a healthy aspect but, in the case of an animal in gestational state, brucellosis is the cause of abortions, sterility, infertility or mastitis. This bacterium is spread in the environment by the infected animals and survives in the ground and in all organic matter (placenta, amniotic liquid and other fluids eliminated during birth of animals). It is very resistant to desiccation, which contributes to its viable permanence for a long time (months) in the straw and dust of stables, in manure, and in homemade dairy products such as milk, butter and unpasteurized cheeses.

How is Brucellosis Transmitted?

In towns, the main vehicle that leads to epidemic outbreaks is consumption of unpasteurized milk, butter manufactured with said milk and homemade cheeses (urban–alimentary transmission).

In rural environments, man acquires the bacteria through direct contact with infected animals giving birth (veterinarians, rural workers) through contact with its excretas or abortion waste by-products—dust, hair, or contaminated facilities—and through eroded skin or splashes affecting eyes. People in charge of milking, shepherds, cowhands or people who live in contact with animals have the greater infection risks; butchers who manipulate infected tissues and viscera run great risks, and personnel working in laboratories that produce the vaccines and *Brucella* antigens, as well as vaccinators, infect themselves by inhaling aerosols, by accidental inoculation or by blood splatter. Even in very cold climates, the ground where births have taken place allows the bacteria to survive for several months, and whoever inhales aerosols (workers or visitors) may get ill.

What are Human Brucellosis Symptoms?

The symptoms are very high fever with "feverish chills" or shivers; abundant sudoration, physical weakness, or intense joint and muscular pains. It can also cause testicle infection. Bone affectation is usual. The most frequent are *sacroileítis* in young people and *espondilitis* in elderly men.

Who is at Risk?

It represents a professional risk among shepherds, abattoir workers, butchers (due to hand microtrauma), workers of dairy or meat processing plants, veterinarians, wool or leather industries workers, laboratory workers, and stable cleaning workers (due to aerosols).

HOW IS BRUCELLOSIS PREVENTED?

The following measures are indispensable for preventing animal brucellosis in rural environments:

- Train personnel in the farm to inform about sick animals.
- Daily inspection of animals.
- Use rubber gloves and safety goggles; use protective cover gear for injuries while handling domestic animals, including its secretions, excretions and skeletons.
- Immediately and adequately sacrifice terminally sick animals, withdrawing them from the premises.
- Perform autopsies on animals that died for unknown reasons.
- Carry on animal vaccination programs.
- Avoid shared ventilation and direct contact with other animals.
- Put under quarantine animals recently introduced in a flock.
- Use different buckets for food and for collecting manure.

For avoiding human brucellosis:

- Know the transmission routes and formulate a strategy capable of minimizing the risk of acquiring the disease.
- Visitors to a farm where animals have given birth are exposed to aerosols of the environment dust, which contains the bacteria;: many have become infected with brucellosis in this way. A few minutes are enough to become infected.
- Dangerous food: unpasteurized dairy foods.

REFERENCES

Troncoso, A.; Bär, N. Food-borne diseases. How to prevent diseases transmitted by food, Buenos Aires, Rene Baron Foundation, 2011.

Troncoso, A; Ruthanne, C. Outbreak Foodborne disease, Buenos Aires, Socrate eds, 2012.

Troncoso, A; Garcia-Moreno, I. The danger of underestimating the risks related to the consumption of contaminated food, Buenos Aires, Cuentahilos eds, 2011.

Chapter 8

TOXOPLASMOSIS

Between 30 and 65% of the world population is considered to be infected by this disease transmitted through kittens. Given that raw or insufficiently cooked red meat is associated with this disease, toxoplasmosis distribution is universal. This infection is habitually asymptomatic and in our country nearly 50% of women arrive to their fertile age without having previously acquired the disease; if infection happens during pregnancy, there exists a serious risk of fetal infection.

WHAT IS TOXOPLASMOSIS?

- Toxoplasmosisis is an infection produced by *Toxoplasma gondii*, a unicellular or single-cell microscopic parasite. Kittens are the infection reservoirs in nature and in the lapse of one to two weeks eliminate parasitic infective microorganisms; this occurs only once in the life of cats and does not infect them.

HOW IS HUMAN TOXOPLASMOSIS ACQUIRED?

1. By digestive route.
- Through raw fruits and vegetables contaminated with cats' fecal matter as cats eliminate the parasite when infected (before they are one year old).

- Through consumption of red meat (beef, pork, lamb).

2. Transplacentary: from mother to fetus.
- It may appear during pregnancy, if the expectant mother does not have antibodies (IgG negative for *Toxoplasma gondii*), due to not having previously acquired the infection.
- If when getting pregnant women already have antibodies, they are immune (they acquired parasite in their childhood or adolescence and are exempt from congenital toxoplasmosis risks). Fetal infection will only appear if *during pregnancy the expectant mother acquires the infection.*

WHAT SYMPTOMS DOES TOXOPLASMOSIS PRESENT?

When toxoplasmosis is acquired in childhood, it is generally benign and does not leave sequelae; it is usually asymptomatic or causes fever and inflamed nodes.

Women who acquire the infection during pregnancy are at risk of transmitting it to the fetus, and the fetus can be born healthy or infected; there exist four degrees of congenital infection:

1) Infection with no clinical manifestations
2) Slight infection, affects sight
3) Serious infection, affects sight and brain
4) Fatal infection

However, a pregnant woman has habitually no symptoms; if she has any symptoms, they are similar to those caused by flu. If the woman has had the infection before her pregnancy, her baby is not at risk, as she has already been exposed to toxoplasmosis and has produced antibodies even if she contracts the infection again; maternal infections during pregnancy do not represent risks for the maternal-fetal-placental-unit.

INFLUENCE OF TOXOPLASMOSIS ON PREGNANCY

1) Non-infected newborn baby.
2) Intrauterine death.

3) Premature labor.
4) Prematurity.
5) Fatal infection:

- Brain and/or eye damage
- Intracranial calcifications
- Hydrocephaly—maturation delay

6) Persistent postnatal infection without evident disease.
There is a reverse correlation between gestational age and fetopathy severity:
The lower the gestational age, the greater the fetal infection severity.

The more precocious the maternal infection is, the more severe the fetopathy is.

There is no correlation between the maternal infection benignancy and the fetal disease severity.

WHO ARE THOSE AT RISK?

It is important to distinguish which women arrive to fertile age and may have toxoplasmic infection; it must be detected which women in fertile age are seronegative (IgG antitoxoplasma antibodies) = SUSCEPTIBLE of contracting infection by not having antibodies. *They are the population at risk.*

DOCUMENTED RISK FACTORS: IN ACCORDANCE WITH THEIR ORDER OF IMPORTANCE

1) Insufficiently cooked beef intake.
2) Cross contamination: infrequent knife washing while preparing beef.
3) Cat litter tray incorrectly cleaned.
4) Insufficiently cooked lamb and/or pork intake.
5) Raw fruits and vegetables intake.

WHAT ARE THE PREVENTION MEASURES?

- Avoid raw or badly cooked meats and cover hands for its manipulation.
- Avoid eating raw fruits and vegetables not prepared at home. In those prepared at home, take care in washing fruits and vegetables.
- Cat litter should be eliminated daily.
- If the pregnant woman has had no contact with the parasite, if she has cats that are not kittens, and if they are kittens, the pregnant woman should avoid picking up fecal matter. She should not carry on gardening activities.
- Take into account basic hygiene measures: such as washing hands, washing foods and kitchen utensils and washing the pet's utensils (cats).

ALL THIS IS NEEDED FOR CONTRACTING THE INFECTION THROUGH THE CAT

- That this is the first time in its life that the cat is infected.
- That no more than three weeks have elapsed since the infection occurred.
- That feces are left in the litter for more than 24 hours.
- That feces are touched with bare hands.
- That without having washed his/her hands, the person touches his/her mouth.
- That the person has never being infected before (susceptible).

The most dangerous habit: carnivorism

Vegetarians are not free from toxoplasmosis risk.

REFERENCES

Troncoso, A; Garcia-Moreno, I. The danger of underestimating the risks related to the consumption of contaminated food, Buenos Aires, Cuentahilos eds, 2011.

Troncoso, A; Ruthanne, C. Outbreak Foodborne disease, Buenos Aires, Socrate eds, 2012.

Troncoso, A ; Baron AP. Toxi-Infection Alimentaire-Risques sanitaires liés à l'eau et à l'alimentation.Le livre que vous ne pouvez pas vous premettre d'ignorer, Buenos Aires, Socrate eds, 2012.

INDEX